REBECCA VAN VLIET

Fuel for Life

Plant-based foods and their benefits

"Dedicate yourself to continuous personal improvement you are your most precious resource."

-BRIAN TRACEY

Contents

1

Introduction

What is the definition of plant-based eating?

Plant-based eating refers to a dietary approach that primarily focuses on eating foods derived from plants, such as fruits, vegetables, whole grains, nuts, seeds, and legumes, while minimizing or excluding animal products. The emphasis is on plant-derived sources for obtaining nutrients and energy.

The motivation for choosing plant-based eating can include health reasons, environmental concerns, and ethical considerations related to animal welfare. Studies suggest that a well-balanced plant-based diet can provide the necessary nutrients for overall health and may be associated with various health benefits, including a reduced risk of chronic diseases.

In recent years, there has been a growing awareness of the health benefits associated with plant-based eating. As individuals seek to enhance their well-being and make conscious choices about their diets, the focus on incorporating more plant-based foods has gained popularity. In this book, we will explore a diverse range of nutritious plant-based foods that not only contribute to overall health but also add a delightful array of colors, flavors, and textures to your meals.

2

Food Groups

Fruits

Apple
  Apricot
  Avocado
  Banana
  Blackberry
  Blueberry
  Cantaloupe
  Cherry
  Clementine
  Cranberry
  Date
  Dragon fruit
  Elderberry
  Fig
Grape
  Grapefruit

Guava
Lemon
Lychee
 Mango
Nectarine
 Orange
 Papaya
Passion fruit
Peach
Pear
Pineapple
Plum
Pomegranate
Star fruit
 Strawberry
 Tangerine
 Watermelon

The nutritional value of fruits can vary widely depending on the specific type of fruit.

Here are some general nutritional components commonly found in fruits:

1. **Vitamins**: Fruits are rich in various vitamins, including vitamin C, vitamin A, vitamin K, and B vitamins.
2. **Minerals**: Fruits contain essential minerals such as potassium, magnesium, and folate.
3. **Dietary Fiber**: Fruits are a good source of dietary fiber, which

is important for digestive health. Fiber can help regulate bowel movements and contribute to a feeling of fullness.

4. **Antioxidants**: Many fruits are packed with antioxidants, such as flavonoids and polyphenols, which help protect the body's cells from damage caused by free radicals.
5. **Natural Sugars**: Fruits contain natural sugars, primarily fructose, which provide a source of energy. The fiber content in fruits helps slow down the absorption of sugars, providing a more stable energy release.
6. **Water**: Fruits have high water content, contributing to hydration and helping to maintain overall fluid balance in the body.
7. **Calories**: Fruits are low in calories, making them a healthy and nutritious snack option.

Here is a brief overview of the nutritional content of some common fruits:

Apples: Are a good source of fiber and vitamin C.

Bananas: High in potassium, vitamin B6, and provide a quick energy boost.

Oranges: Rich in vitamin C, fiber, and various antioxidants.

Berries (Strawberries, Blueberries, Raspberries): High in vitamins, antioxidants, and fiber.

Mangoes: Rich in vitamin C, vitamin A, and potassium.

Grapes: Contain antioxidants and vitamin C.

Watermelon: High water content, are a good source of vitamin C and antioxidants.

Vegetables

Asparagus
Bell pepper
Broccoli
Brussels sprouts
Cabbage
Carrot
Cauliflower
Celery
Corn
Cucumber
Eggplant
Garlic
Green beans
Kale
Lettuce
Mushrooms
Onions
Peas
Potato
Pumpkin
Radish
Spinach
Squash
Tomato
Turnip
Yam
Zucchini

The nutritional value of vegetables varies widely depending on the specific type of vegetable.

Here are some general nutritional components commonly found in vegetables.

1. **Vitamins**: Vegetables are rich in various vitamins, including vitamin A, vitamin C, vitamin K, and various B vitamins.
2. **Minerals**: Vegetables provide essential minerals such as potassium, magnesium, calcium, and iron.
3. **Dietary Fiber**: Vegetables are an excellent source of dietary fiber, which is crucial for digestive health, regulating blood sugar levels, and supporting a feeling of fullness.
4. **Antioxidants**: Many vegetables contain antioxidants , flavoring, and polyphenols, which help protect the body's cells from oxidative stress.
5. **Nutrients**: Vegetables often contain phytonutrients, plant compounds that may have various health benefits, including anti-inflammatory and immune-boosting properties.
6. **Low in Calories**: Most vegetables are low in calories, making them a nutrient-dense option for those looking to maintain a healthy weight.

Here is a brief overview of the nutritional content of some common vegetables:

Leafy Greens (Spinach, Kale, Lettuce): High in vitamins A, C, and K, as well as folate and iron.

Broccoli: Rich in vitamins C and K, fiber, and antioxidants.

Carrots: Excellent source of beta-carotene (a form of vitamin A), and a good source of fiber.

Tomatoes: Provide vitamins C and K, as well as antioxidants like lycopene.

Bell Peppers: High in vitamin C, A, and potassium.

Sweet Potatoes: Rich in beta-carotene, vitamin C, and fiber.

Cauliflower: Contains vitamins C & K and is a good source of fiber.

Grains

Barley
  Brown rice
  Buckwheat
  Bulgur
  Chia seeds
  Farro
  Flax seeds
  Millet
  Oats
  Quinoa
  Rye
  Spelt
  Wheat
  Wild rice

The nutritional value of grains can vary significantly depending on the specific type of grain. However, grains, in general, are a good source of carbohydrates, fiber, and various essential nutrients.

Here is a general overview of the nutritional content of some common grains:

Brown Rice: Carbohydrates, Fiber, B vitamins (especially B1, B3, and B6), Magnesium and Iron.

Quinoa: Complete protein (contains all essential amino acids), Carbohydrates, Fiber, B vitamins, Iron and Magnesium.

Oats: Carbohydrates, Soluble fiber, B vitamins, Iron, Magnesium and Zinc.

Barley: Carbohydrates, Fiber, B vitamins, Iron, Magnesium and Selenium.

Buckwheat: Carbohydrates, Fiber, Protein, B vitamins, Iron and Magnesium.

Millet: Carbohydrates, Fiber, B vitamins, Iron and Magnesium.

Wheat (Whole Wheat): Carbohydrates, Fiber, B vitamins (especially B1, B3, and B6), Iron and Magnesium.

Rye: Carbohydrates, Fiber, B vitamins, Iron, Magnesium and Zinc.

Legumes

Black beans
  Black-eyed peas
  Butter beans
  Cannellini beans
  Chickpeas

Chickpea flour
Edamame
Fava beans
Garbanzo beans
Great Northern beans
Kidney beans
Lentils
Lima beans
Mung beans
Navy beans
Peanuts
Pinto beans
Soybeans
Split peas

Legumes are highly nutritious and provide a rich source of protein, dietary fiber, vitamins, and minerals.

Here is a general overview of the nutritional content of common legumes:

Lentils: Protein, Dietary fiber, Folate,Iron, Potassium, Vitamin B1 (Thiamine)

Chickpeas (Garbanzo beans): Protein, Dietary fiber, Folate,Iron, Magnesium and Vitamin B6.

Black beans: Protein, Dietary fiber, Folate, Iron, Magnesium and Potassium.

Kidney beans: Protein, Dietary fiber, Folate, Iron, Magnesium and Potassium.

Navy beans: Protein, Dietary fiber, Folate,Iron, Magnesium and Potassium.

Pinto beans: Protein, Dietary fiber, Folate, Iron,Magnesium and Potassium.

Lima beans: Protein, Dietary fiber, Folate,Iron, Magnesium and Potassium.

Cannellini beans: Protein, Dietary fiber, Folate, Iron,Magnesium and Potassium.

Fava beans: Protein, Dietary fiber, Folate, Iron,Magnesium and Potassium.

Split peas (green and yellow): Protein, Dietary fiber, Folate,Iron, Magnesium and Potassium.

Black-eyed peas: Protein, Dietary fiber, Folate, Iron,Magnesium and Potassium.

Mung beans: Protein, Dietary fiber, Folate, Iron, Magnesium and Potassium.

Soybeans: Protein (complete protein source), Dietary fiber, Folate,Iron, Magnesium and Potassium.

Edamame: Protein, Dietary fiber, Folate,Iron, Magnesium and Potassium.

Peanuts: Protein, Dietary fiber, Folate, Iron, Magnesium and Potassium.

Nuts and Seeds

Nuts:

Almonds
Brazil nuts
Cashews
Chestnuts
Hazelnuts
Macadamia nuts
Peanuts
Pecans
Pine nuts
Pistachios
Walnuts

Seeds:
Chia seeds
Flax seeds
Hemp seeds
Pumpkin seeds
Sesame seed
Sunflower seeds
Poppy seeds
Quinoa

Nuts and seeds are nutrient-dense foods that offer a variety of health benefits.

Here is a general overview of the nutritional content of common nuts and seeds:

Nuts

Almonds: Healthy monounsaturated fats, Protein, Fiber, Vitamin E, Magnesium and Calcium.

Brazil nuts: Selenium (high levels), Healthy fats, Protein and Fiber.

Cashews: Healthy monounsaturated fats, Protein, Copper, Iron and Magnesium.

Chestnuts: Low in fat compared to other nuts, Rich in vitamin C and Good source of dietary fiber

Hazelnut: Healthy monounsaturated fats, Protein, Fiber, Vitamin E and Magnesium.

Macadamia nuts: Healthy monounsaturated fats, Low in Omega-6 fatty acids, Thiamine (B1) and Manganese.

Peanuts: Protein, Healthy monounsaturated and polyunsaturated fats, Niacin (B3), Folate and Magnesium.

Pecans: Healthy monounsaturated fats, Protein, Fiber, Thiamine (B1) and Zinc.

Pine nuts: Healthy monounsaturated fats, Protein, Vitamin K, Magnesium and Zinc.

Pistachios: Healthy monounsaturated fats, Protein, Fiber, Vitamin B6 and Phosphorus.

Walnuts: Omega-3 fatty acids, Protein, Fiber, Antioxidants and Vitamin E.

Seeds

Chia seeds: Omega-3 fatty acids, Fiber, Protein, Calcium and Phosphorus.

Flaxseeds: Omega-3 fatty acids (alpha-linolenic acid), Fiber, Protein and Lignans (antioxidants).

Hemp seeds: Omega-3 and Omega-6 fatty acids, Protein (complete protein source), Fiber, Vitamin E and Magnesium.

Pumpkin seeds (Pepitas): Protein, Healthy fats, Magnesium, Iron and Zinc.

Sesame seeds: Protein, Healthy monounsaturated and polyunsaturated fats,Fiber, Calcium, and Iron.

Sunflower seeds: Protein, Healthy fats, Vitamin E, Selenium and Magnesium.

Poppy seeds: Protein, Healthy fats, Calcium, Iron and Magnesium.

Quinoa: Complete protein (contains all essential amino acids), Carbohydrates, Fiber, Iron and Magnesium.

Including a variety of nuts and seeds in your day can provide essential nutrients, contribute to heart health, and offer numerous other health benefits. However, it is important to be mindful of portion sizes due to their calorie density.

Plant-Based Milks

Plant-based milk alternatives have become increasingly popular, providing options for individuals who are lactose intolerant, allergic to dairy, or following a vegan or plant-based eating.

Here is a list of some common plant-based milk alternatives:

Almond Milk: Made from almonds, it has a mild, slightly nutty flavor.
Soy Milk: Made from whole soybeans, it has a creamy texture and is a good source of protein.
Oat Milk: Made from whole oats, it has a naturally sweet flavor and a creamy consistency.

Coconut Milk: Made from the liquid extracted from coconut flesh, it has a rich and tropical taste.

Rice Milk: Made from brown rice, it has a neutral flavor and is often slightly sweeter than other alternatives.

Cashew Milk: Made from cashews, it has a creamy texture and a mild, slightly sweet taste.

Hemp Milk: Made from hemp seeds, it has a nutty flavor and provides a good source of **omega-3 fatty acids**.

Flax Milk: Made from flax seeds, it has a mild, slightly nutty taste and is often enriched with nutrients like **calcium and vitamin D**.

Pea Milk: Made from yellow peas, it has a neutral taste and is a good source of **protein**.

Quinoa Milk: Made from quinoa, it has a mild, slightly nutty flavor and is often fortified with nutrients.

Macadamia Milk: Made from macadamia nuts, it has a rich and creamy texture with a subtle nutty flavor.

Hazelnut Milk: Made from hazelnuts, it has a distinct hazelnut flavor and is often sweetened.

Walnut Milk: Made from walnuts, it has a mild, slightly earthy flavor and is rich in **omega-3 fatty acids**.

Sunflower Seed Milk: Made from sunflower seeds, it has a nutty taste and is a good source of **vitamin E**.

Pistachio Milk: Made from pistachios, it has a unique pistachio flavor and is often creamy.

It is important to note that the nutritional content, taste, and texture can vary between brands and varieties of plant-based milk. Additionally, many plant-based milks are fortified with vitamins and minerals such as calcium and vitamin D to mimic the nutritional profile of cow's milk. When choosing a plant-based milk, it is a good idea to check the product's label for fortification and choose options that suit your taste preferences and nutritional needs.

Healthy Fats

Plant-based fats are a key component of a healthy, balanced diet, and they offer various health benefits.

Here is a list of healthy plant-based fats that you can include in your day:

Avocado: Rich in monounsaturated fats, High in fiber, vitamins, and minerals

Nuts: Almonds, Brazil nuts, Cashews, Hazelnuts, Pecans, Pistachios and Walnuts.

Seeds: Chia seeds, Flax seeds, Pumpkin seeds (pepitas), Sesame seeds and Sunflower seeds.

Nut and Seed Butters: Almond butter, Peanut butter (choose varieties without added sugars and oils) and Sunflower seed butter.

Soy: Tofu and Tempeh are sources of plant-based fats, Edamame (young soybeans)

Hemp Seeds: Rich in omega-3 and omega-6 fatty acids, a good source of protein and minerals.

Chia Seeds: High in omega-3 fatty acids and an excellent source of fiber.

Pumpkin Seed Oil: Contains a good balance of omega-3 and omega-6 fatty acids.

Seaweed: Some seaweed varieties, like nori, contain healthy fats, a good source of minerals and antioxidants.

Oils and butters have been removed from this list, due to the high saturated fat content. If you want to use oils, please use them in moderation.

1 tablespoon of oil = 120 calories of pure fat, the fiber and nutrients have been stripped away. Where one tablespoon of flax seed =37 calories. Eat olives, not olive oil, eat avocados not avocado oil, eat flax seed, not flax seed oil. Oil can also cause inflammation in your body.

It is also crucial to maintain a balance between several types of fats in your meals. A well-rounded diet that includes a variety of healthy fats can contribute to heart health, brain function, hormone production, and overall well-being.

Spices

Spices are plant-derived and can add flavor, aroma, and nutritional benefits to a variety of plant-based dishes. They are an excellent way to enhance the taste of your meals.

Common plant-based spices include:

Basil
Black pepper
Cayenne pepper
Chives
Cinnamon
Cloves
Coriander

Cumin

Dill

Garlic

Ginger

Mint

Onion

Oregano

Paprika

Parsley

Rosemary

Sage

Thyme

Turmeric

These spices can be used to add depth of flavor to various plant-based dishes, from soups and stews to salads and stir-fries. Additionally, many spices offer potential health benefits due to their antioxidant, anti-inflammatory, and antimicrobial properties. It is important to note that while spices contribute to overall health, they are typically consumed in small amounts, so their individual impact may be limited.

Here is a list of health benefits associated with different spices.

Anti-Inflammatory Effects:
Turmeric: Contains curcumin, known for its potent anti-inflammatory properties. It may help reduce inflammation in the body.
Antioxidant Properties:
Cinnamon: High in antioxidants, which can help neutralize free

radicals and reduce oxidative stress in the body.

Cloves: Rich in antioxidants, cloves have been shown to have anti-inflammatory and antimicrobial effects.

Digestive Health:

Ginger: Known for its digestive benefits, ginger may help alleviate nausea, reduce inflammation, and promote overall digestive health.

Heart Health:

Garlic: Studies suggest that garlic may have cardiovascular benefits, including lowering blood pressure and improving cholesterol levels.

Blood Sugar Regulation:

Cumin: Some research indicates that cumin may help improve insulin sensitivity and regulate blood sugar levels.

Immune System Support:

Cayenne Pepper: Contains capsaicin, which has immune-modulating and anti-inflammatory effects.

Cancer Prevention:

Turmeric: Curcumin, found in turmeric, has been studied for its potential role in preventing and treating cancer due to its anti-inflammatory and antioxidant properties.

Weight Management:

Cayenne Pepper: Capsaicin in cayenne pepper may boost metabolism and promote weight loss by increasing calorie expenditure.

3

Implementing Plant-Based Eating

Transitioning to a plant-based diet involves incorporating more plant-derived foods and minimizing or eliminating animal products. Here are some steps to help you implement a plant-based eating approach:

Educate Yourself:

Learn about the benefits of a plant-based diet, nutritional requirements, and potential sources of plant-based protein, iron, calcium, and other essential nutrients.

Familiarize yourself with different plant-based ingredients, recipes, and cooking techniques.

Gradual Transition:

Consider gradually reducing your intake of animal products rather than making an abrupt change. Start by incorporating more plant-based meals into your routine.

Explore Plant-Based Foods:

Experiment with a variety of fruits, vegetables, whole grains, legumes, nuts, and seeds.

Try different plant-based protein sources such as tofu, tempeh, and legumes.

Meal Planning:

Plan your meals in advance to ensure a balanced and varied diet.

Include a mix of vegetables, whole grains, plant-based protein, and healthy fats in each meal.

Cook at Home:

Cooking at home gives you control over ingredients and allows you to experiment with plant-based recipes.

Invest in plant-based cookbooks or explore online resources for inspiration.

Read Labels:

Be mindful of processed foods and check labels for hidden animal products, oils, and sugars.

Look for plant-based alternatives, such as dairy-free milk, plant-based meat substitutes, and egg replacements.

Stay Hydrated:

Drink at least eight cups of water throughout the day.

Consider incorporating herbal teas, infused water, and fresh juices into your beverage choices.

Include Snacks:

Keep a variety of plant-based snacks on hand, such as fresh fruit, raw veggies with hummus, or nuts and seeds.

Explore Ethnic Cuisines:

Many ethnic cuisines have plant-based dishes as staples. Explore

Mediterranean, Asian, and Middle Eastern cuisines for flavorful plant-based options.

Connect with the Plant-Based Community:

Examples: http://simplyplantbasedkitchen.com
http://www.foodhackersclub.com

Consider Supplements:

Depending on your dietary choices, you may need to supplement certain nutrients like vitamin B12, vitamin D, and omega-3 fatty acids.

Listen to Your Body:

Pay attention to how your body responds to the changes. Adjust your meals based on your energy levels, hunger, and overall well-being.

Remember, adopting a plant-based eating approach is a personal journey, and it is okay to take it one step at a time. Make choices that align with your preferences, lifestyle, and health goals.

4

Conclusion

It is never too late to take steps towards better health!

Take it one step at a time. Implementing small changes each month will lead to big changes by the end of the year.

Adopting a plant-based eating approach involves incorporating more plant-derived foods while reducing or eliminating animal products from your diet. This transition offers numerous potential health benefits, including improved heart health, weight management, and a lower risk of chronic diseases. Key steps to implement plant-based eating include educating yourself about nutritional needs, gradually transitioning, exploring diverse plant-based foods, planning meals, cooking at home, reading labels, and connecting with the plant-based community.

It is essential to focus on well-balanced meals that include a variety of fruits, vegetables, whole grains, legumes, nuts, and seeds to ensure you meet your nutritional requirements. Experimenting with different plant-based ingredients, ethnic cuisines, and cooking methods can make the transition enjoyable and sustainable.

Additionally, staying hydrated, considering supplements if necessary, and listening to your body's needs are crucial aspects of a successful plant-based journey.

Remember that the journey toward a plant-based lifestyle is unique for everyone. Whether you choose to fully adopt a plant-based lifestyle or simply incorporate more plant-based meals, making mindful and informed choices will contribute to your overall well-being.

When starting a plant-based lifestyle consult with your healthcare provider, especially if you are on any medications. Your medications may need to be adjusted or stopped.

If you liked this book and have found this information useful, please leave a review.

5

Resources

https://chat.openai.com

http://simplyplantbasedkitchen.com

http://www.foodhackersclub.com